MommyHooray Presents:

The Mental Load

The Invisible Work Behind Everyday Care

by MommyHooray

MommyHooray Presents: The Mental Load
by MommyHooray

Written and published under the pen name MommyHooray.
Illustrations created using digital illustration tools.

Printed in the United States of America.

ISBN: 978-1-972071-40-3

For more stories and updates, visit:
https://sites.google.com/view/mommyhooray/

For the ones who carry the mental load—
the planning, the remembering, the anticipating,
the quiet work that fills every day.

This book is for you.
Your exhaustion has a reason.
Your effort has value.
And the work you do—even when unseen—matters.

With Googolplex Love,

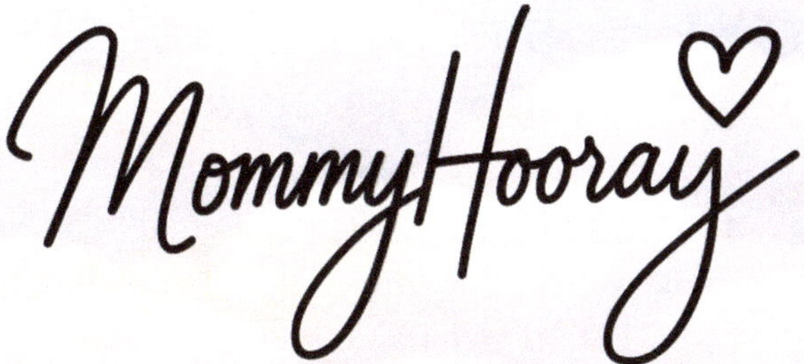

Some work goes unnamed.

You can be exhausted
without anything obvious to point to.

You can be doing so much
and still feel like it doesn't count.

This isn't about productivity
or fixing yourself.

It's about the mental load—
the remembering,
the anticipating,
the invisible holding.

If you've ever felt tired
and couldn't explain why,
there was a reason.

Nothing here needs solving.
What you carry deserves language.

You can lie down and still feel busy.

You can close your eyes and still feel responsible.

Rest doesn't always mean stopping.

Sometimes it means realizing just how much you've been carrying.

I can rest.
My mind can't.

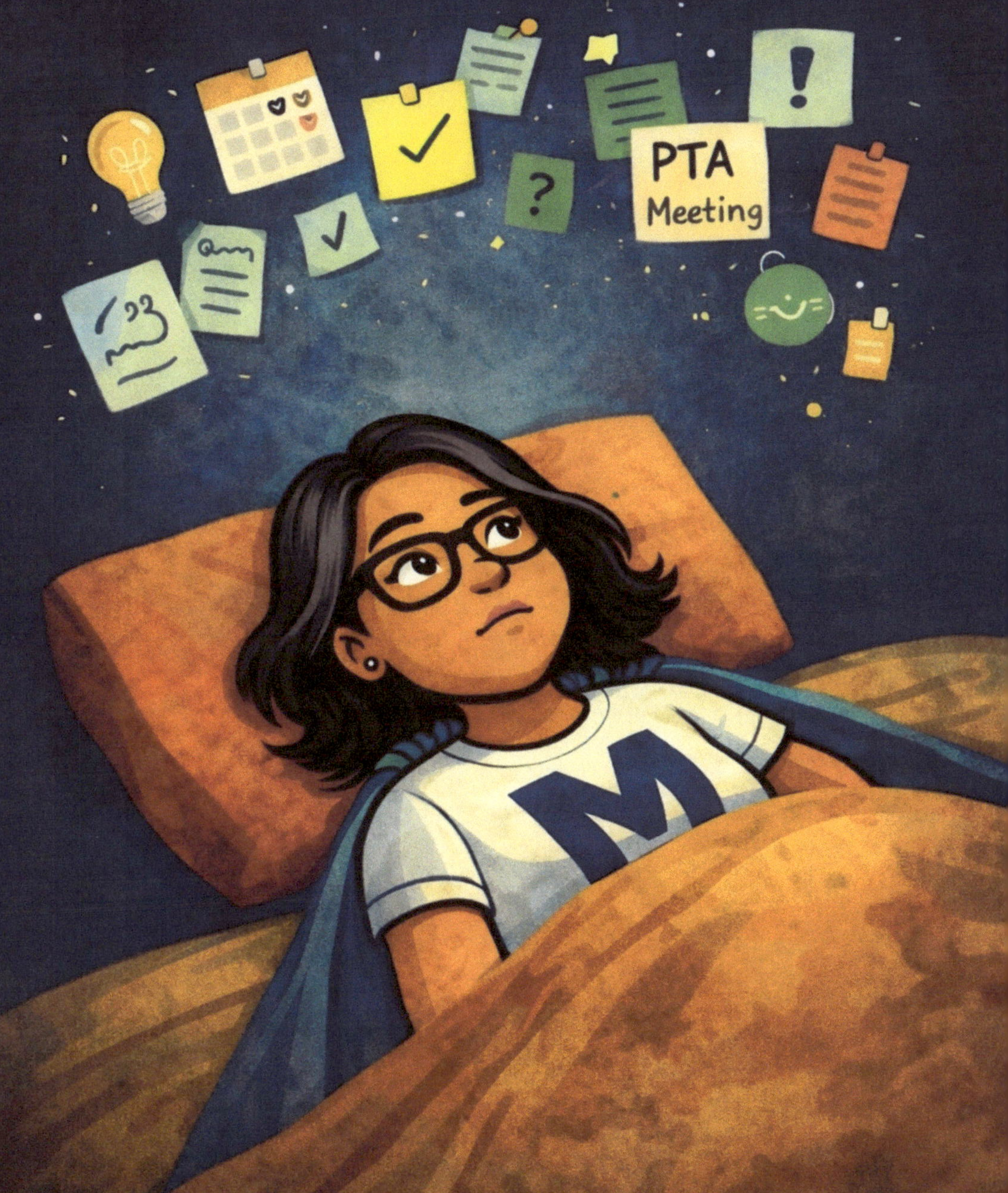

People say asking is easy.

But they don't see the work behind it—
the planning,
the explaining,
the organizing.

Sometimes asking doesn't feel like asking at all.
It feels like another responsibility.

Asking is already another task.

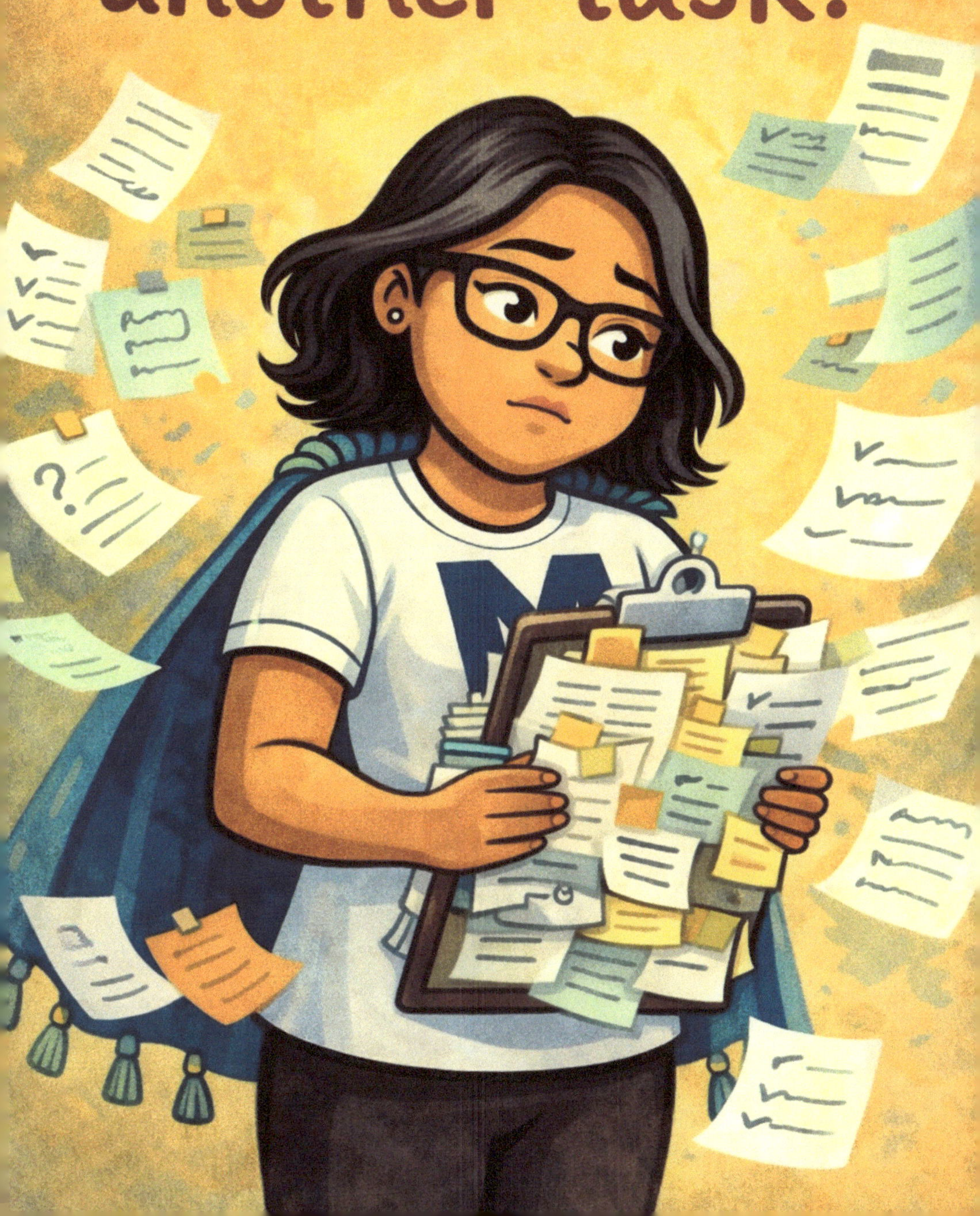

Sitting down doesn’t turn things off.

The remembering keeps going.
The tracking.
The noticing.

The list waits patiently,
quietly continuing in your mind.

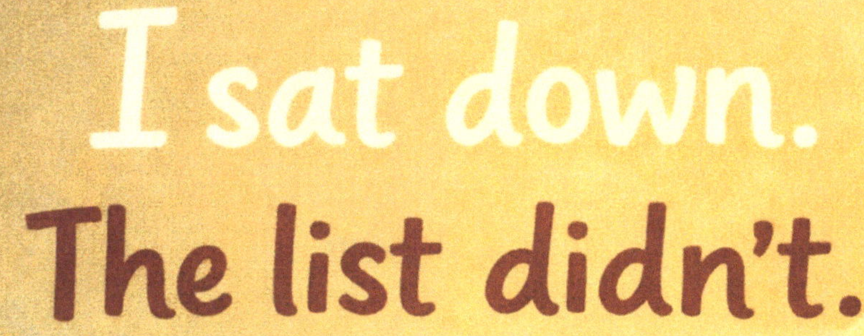
I sat down.
The list didn't.

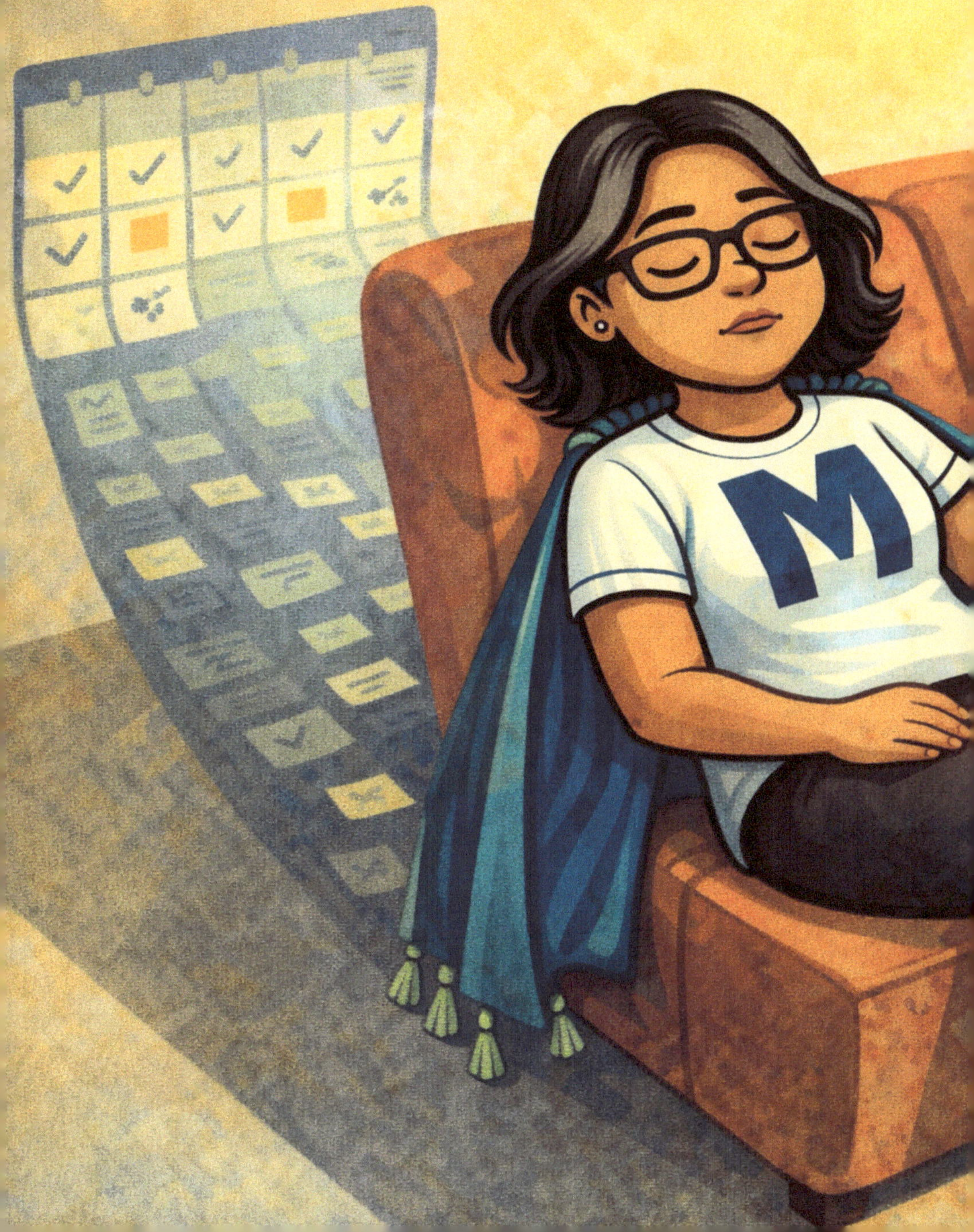

You're not lazy.

You're not bad at coping.

The work you do just doesn't announce itself.

It lives quietly in your head,

holding together the details no one else sees.

Even when it looks like nothing,

you're carrying a lot.

The work you see is only half of it.

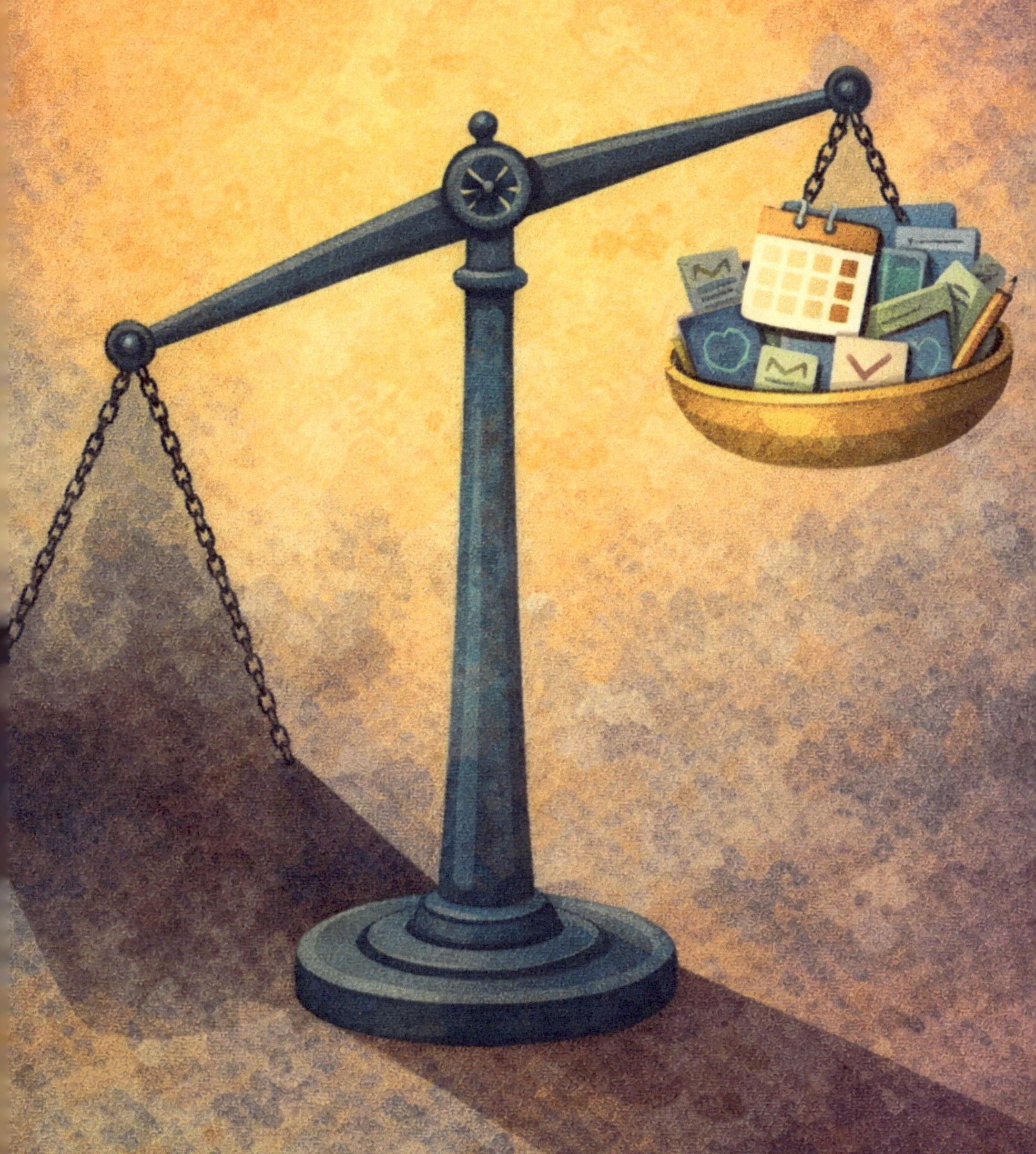

You carry things that don't fit in your hands.

Appointments.

Needs.

What's coming next.

It follows you everywhere,

quietly moving through your day.

And somehow,

you keep it all going.

I carry it everywhere.

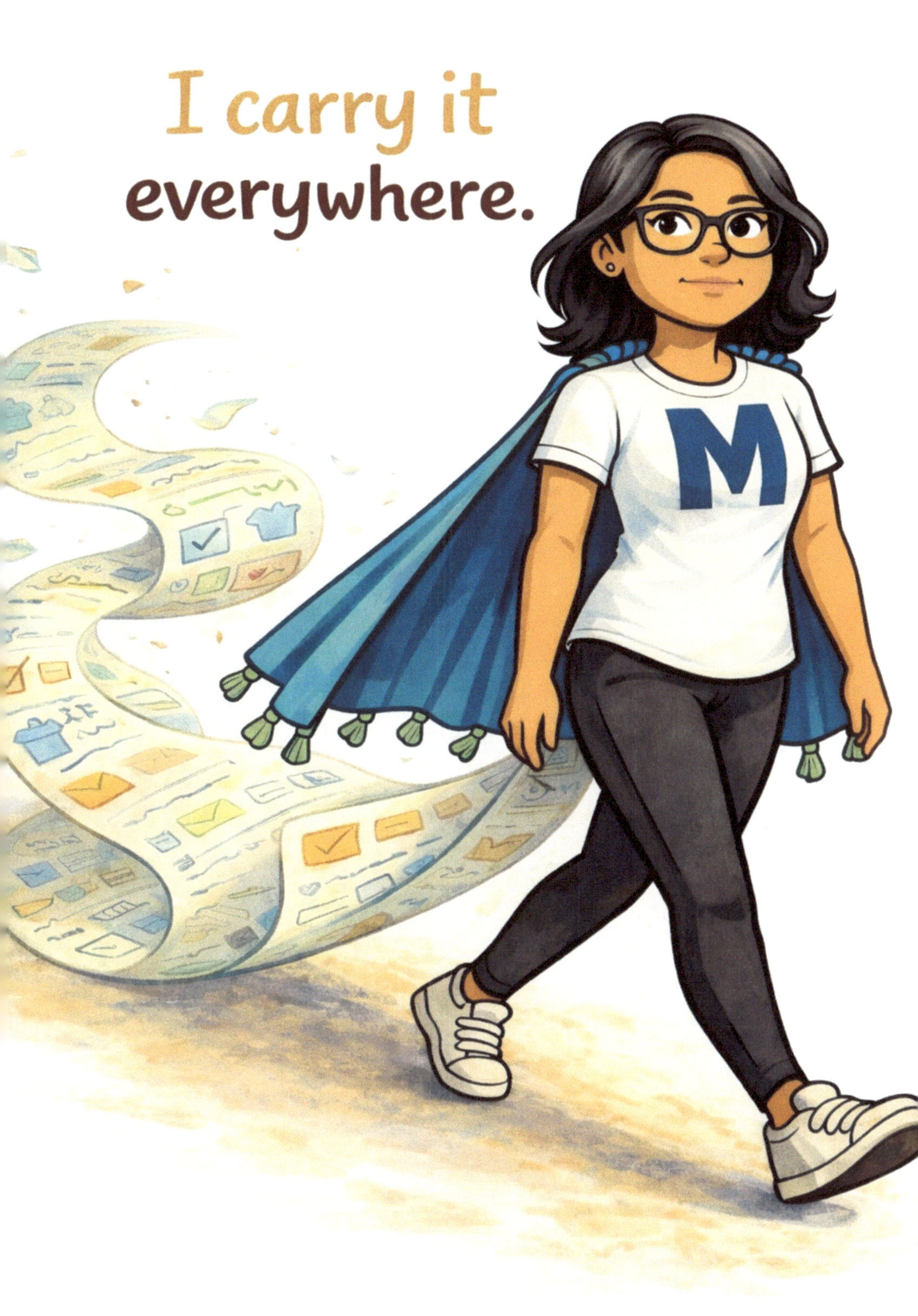

You don't wait for things to fall.

You're already reaching.
Already planning.
Already preventing what hasn't happened yet.

You are always a few steps ahead.

Holding things together
before they even begin to slip.

I'm already thinking three steps ahead.

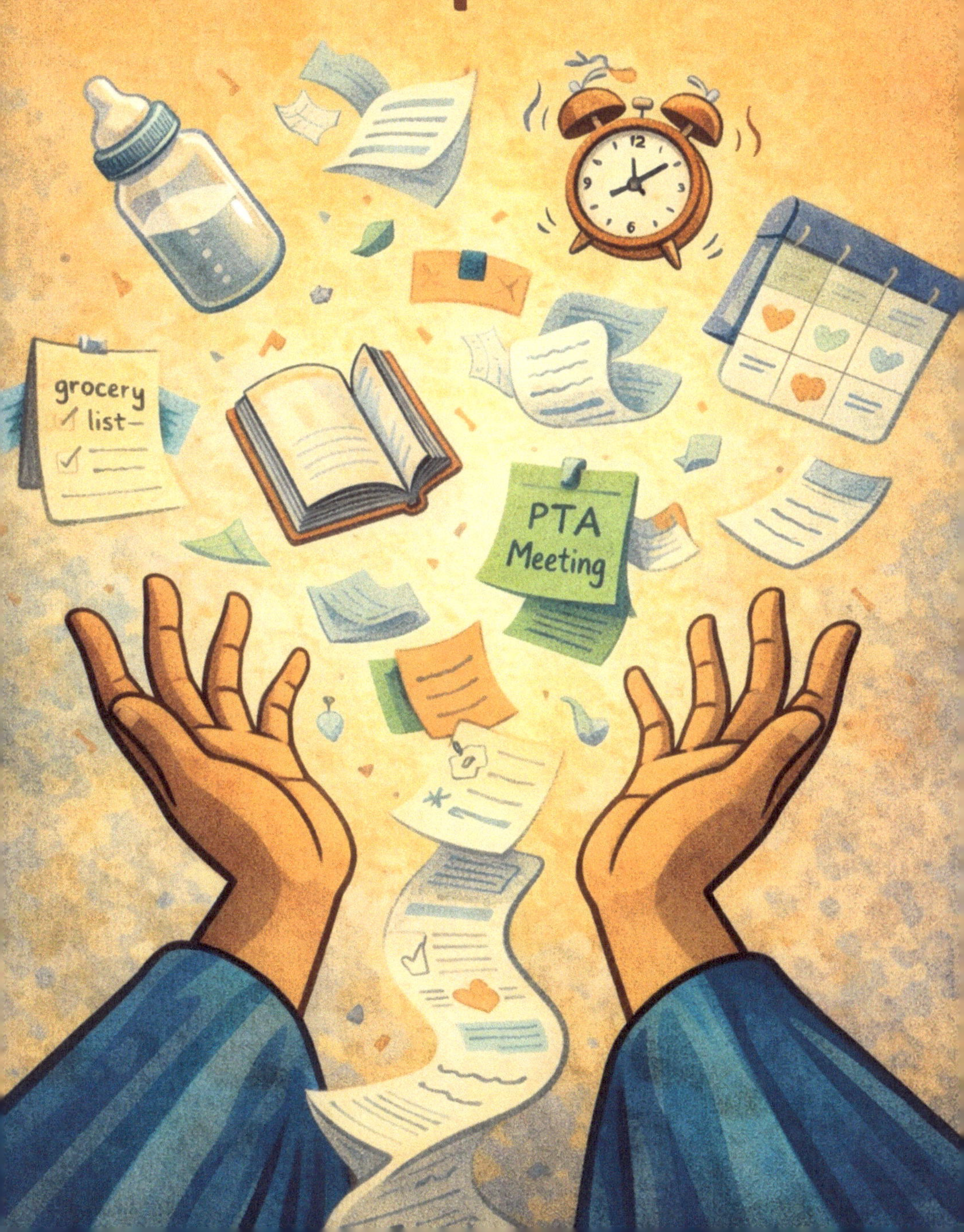

The remembering lands somewhere.

Birthdays.

Forms.

Snacks.

And somehow,
it quietly becomes yours to hold.

Until it feels like it was always yours.

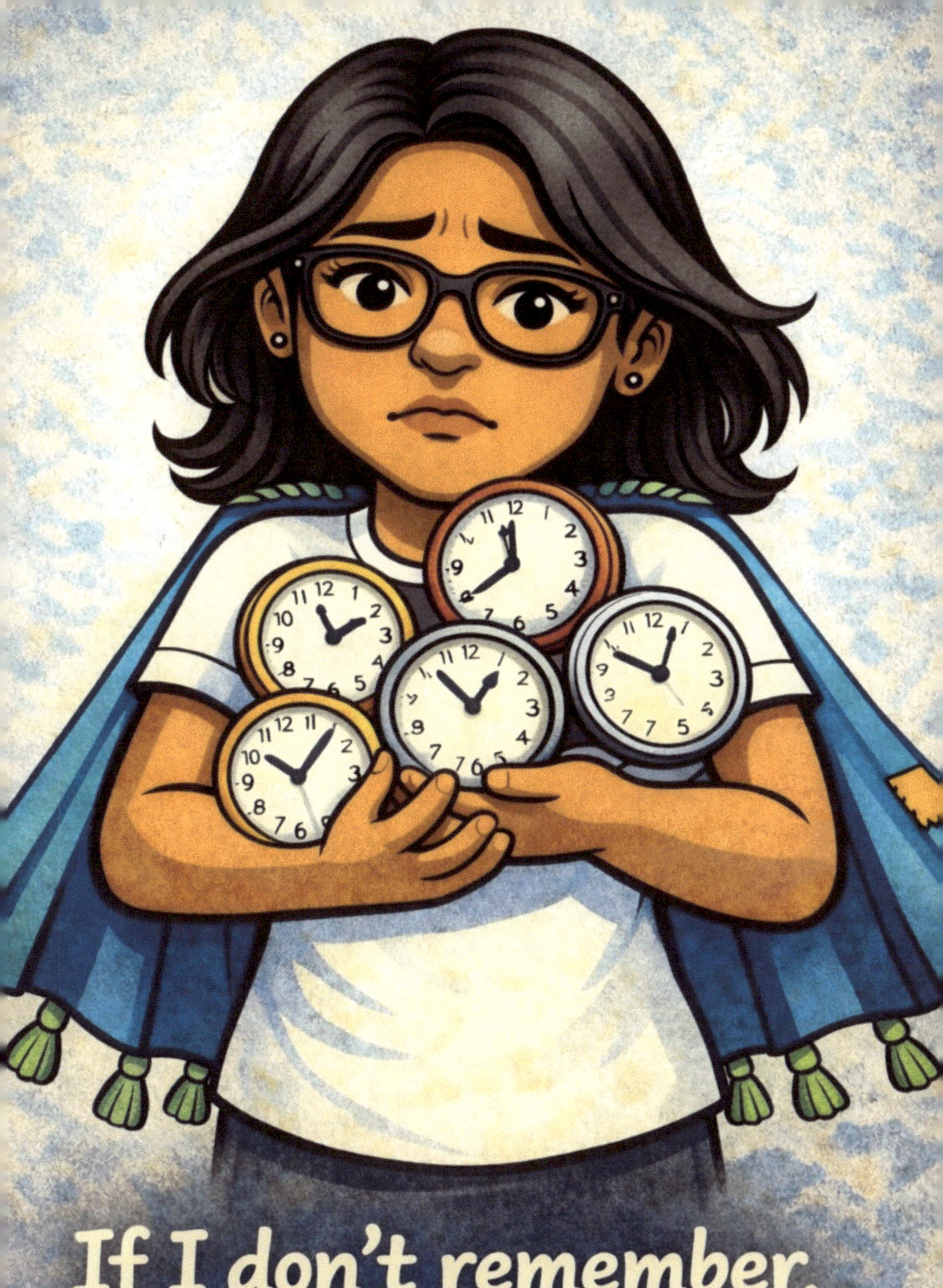

If I don’t remember,
no one does.

You soften the edges.
You absorb the emotions.
You make space so everyone else can land safely.

You hold the moment together,
even when it feels like too much.

That, too, is work.

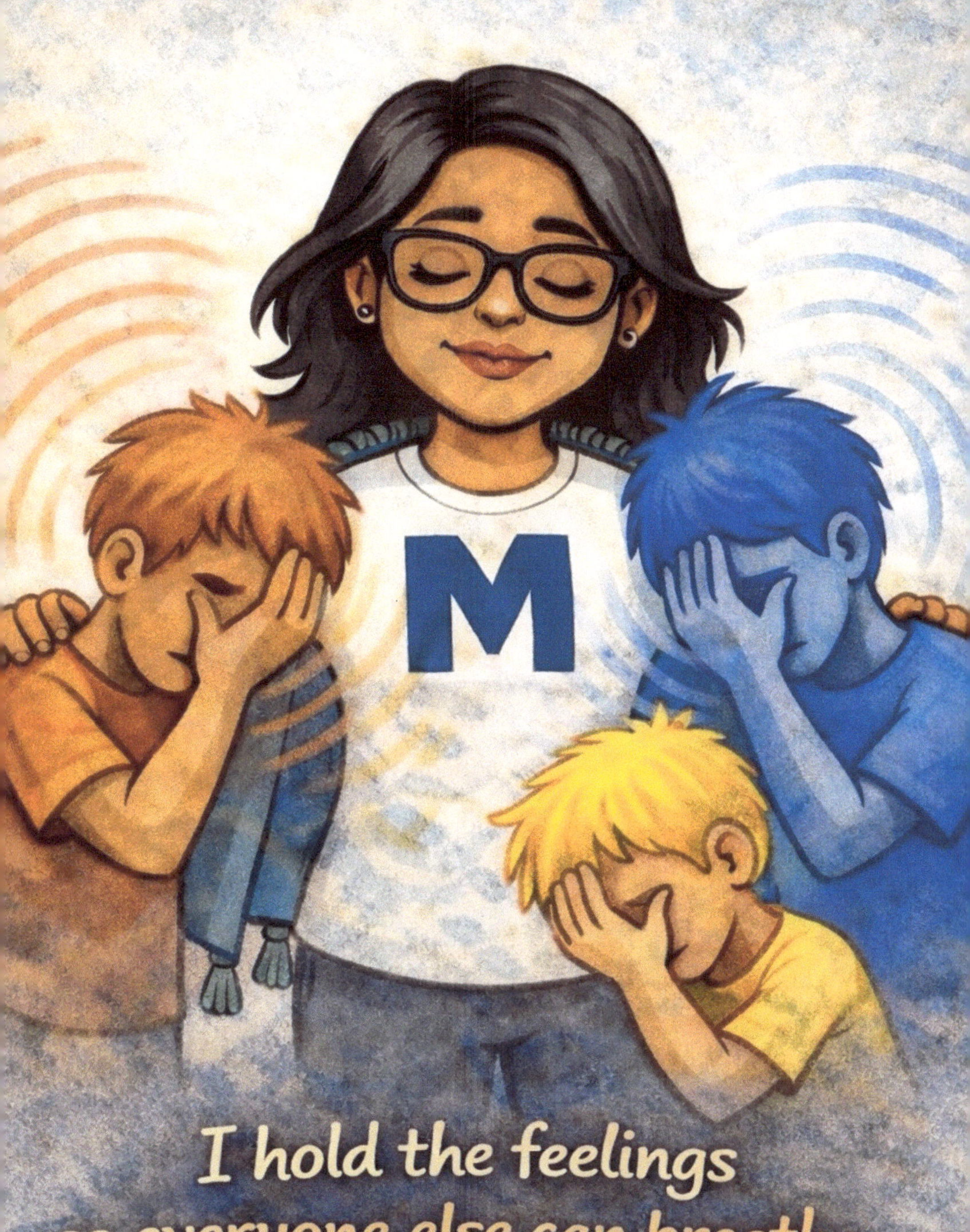
M
I hold the feelings
so everyone else can breathe.

When the house sleeps,
your mind finally has room to speak.

The quiet stretches out around you.
The thoughts you carried all day begin to surface.

This is when the day catches up.

This is when
it gets loud.

People see what's visible.

They notice the things that get finished.

They don't see the rest.

The planning.

The worrying.

The small things you carry in your mind all day.

But you feel it every day.

Invisible work
still has weight.

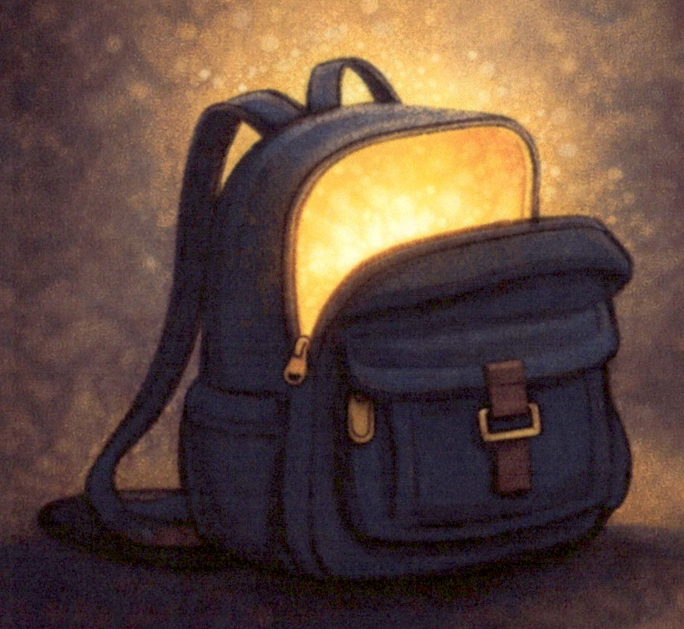

Being needed can feel like love and weight.

It warms your heart.

It sits on your shoulders.

Being needed can fill you.

And sometimes, it can drain you too.

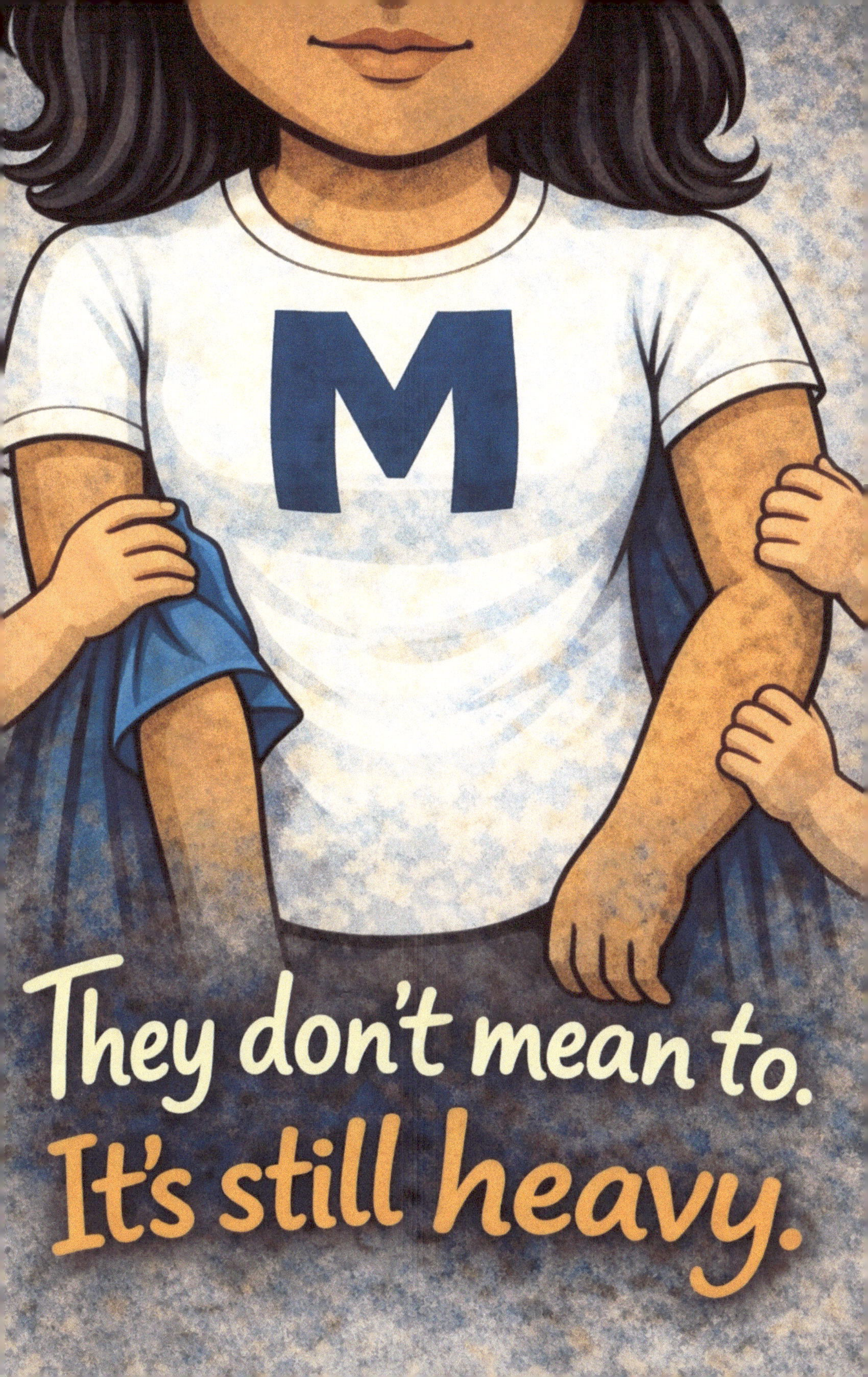
M
They don't mean to.
It's still heavy.

There's no shared calendar for what you hold.
No notification for the weight of it.

It lives in your body.
In your tension.
In your tiredness.

And it follows you into the quiet,
long after everything else is done.

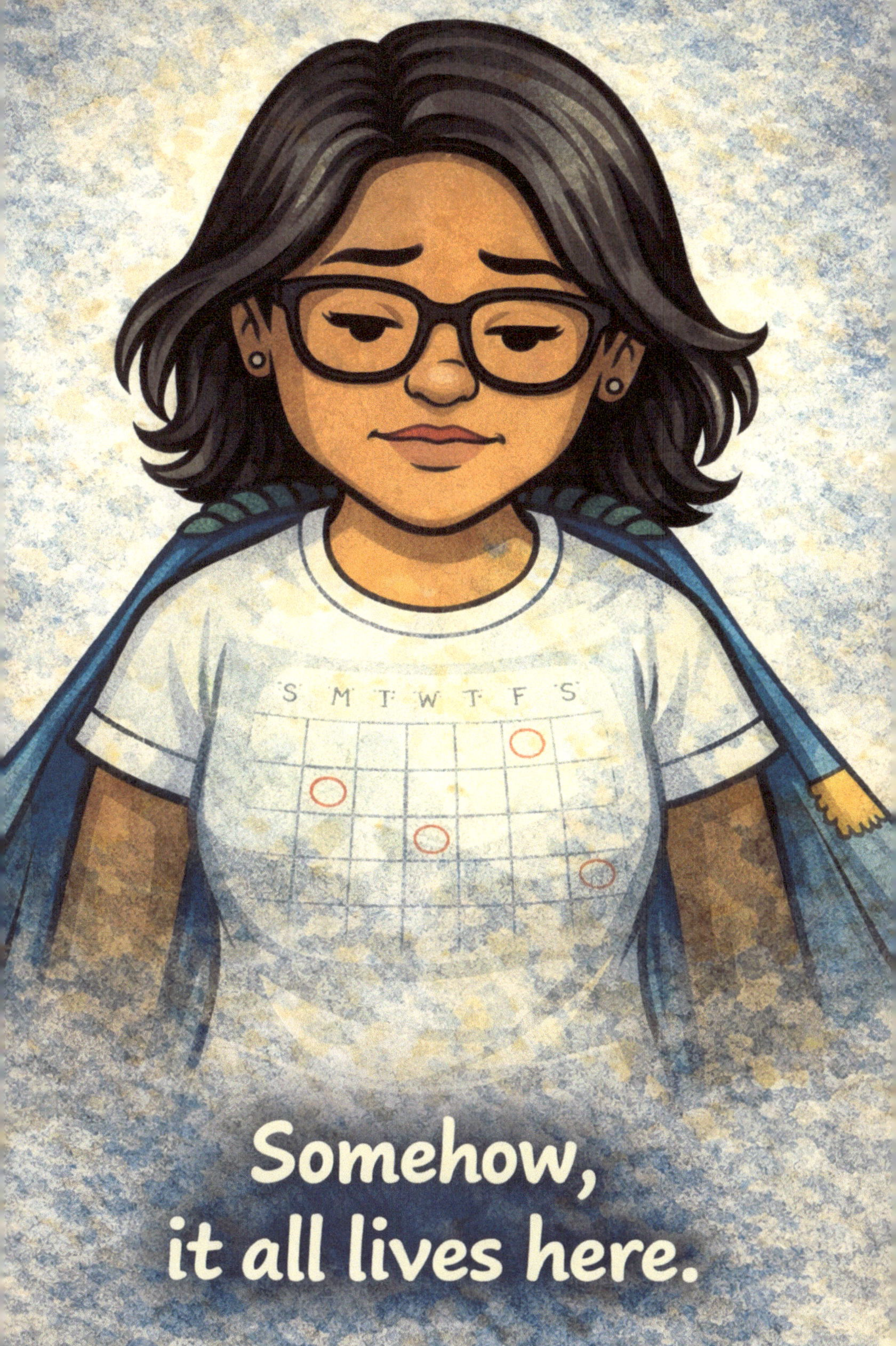

Somehow,
it all lives here.

You wonder why resting didn't seem to fix anything,
and why the tiredness is still there when you wake up.

It's easy to forget that exhaustion
doesn't wait for the right moment to arrive.

And sometimes,
it runs deeper than rest.

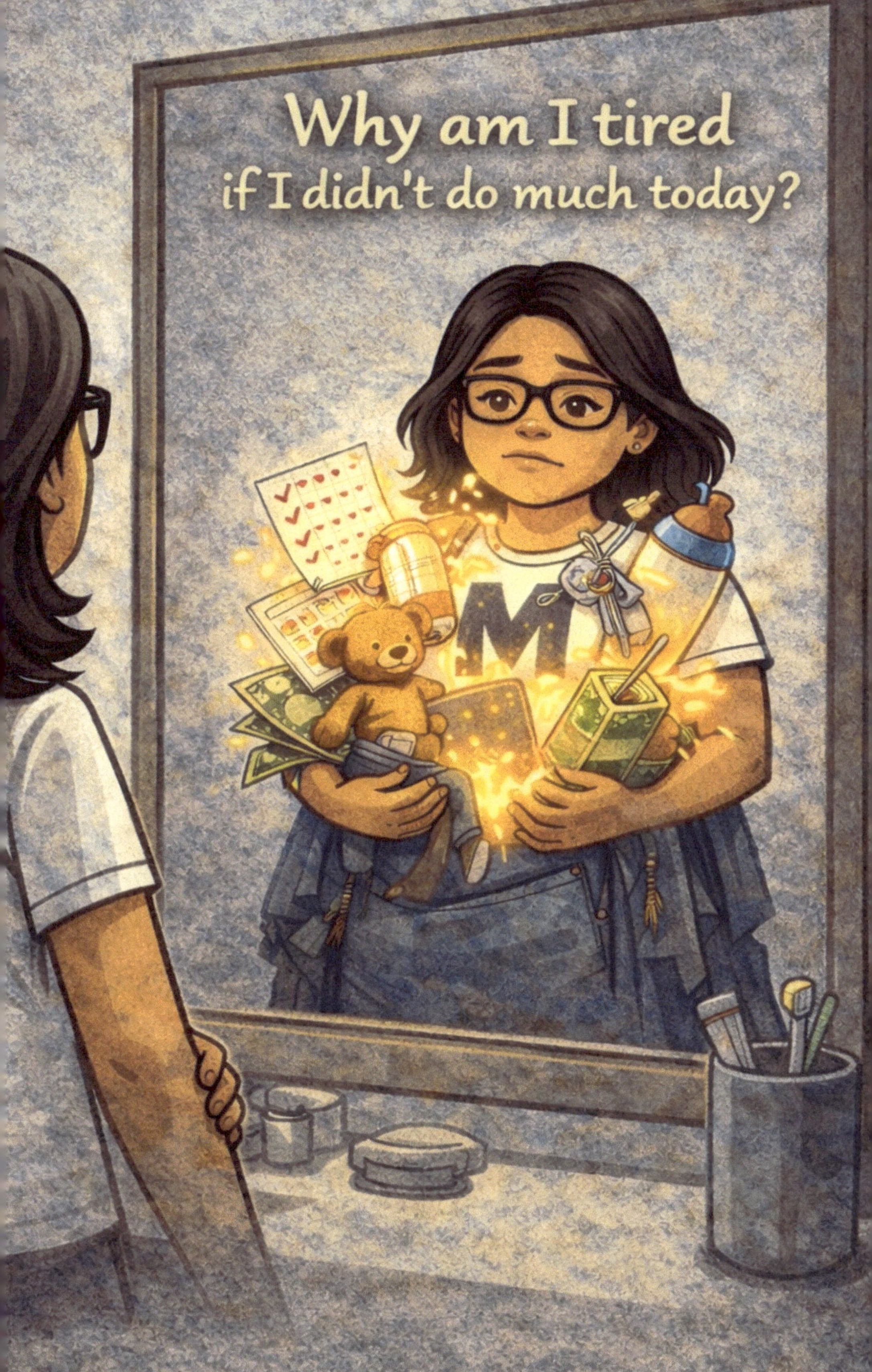
Why am I tired
if I didn't do much today?

Explaining takes energy.
Managing help takes energy.

Sometimes doing it yourself feels easier,
not because it is,
but because you're already carrying everything else.

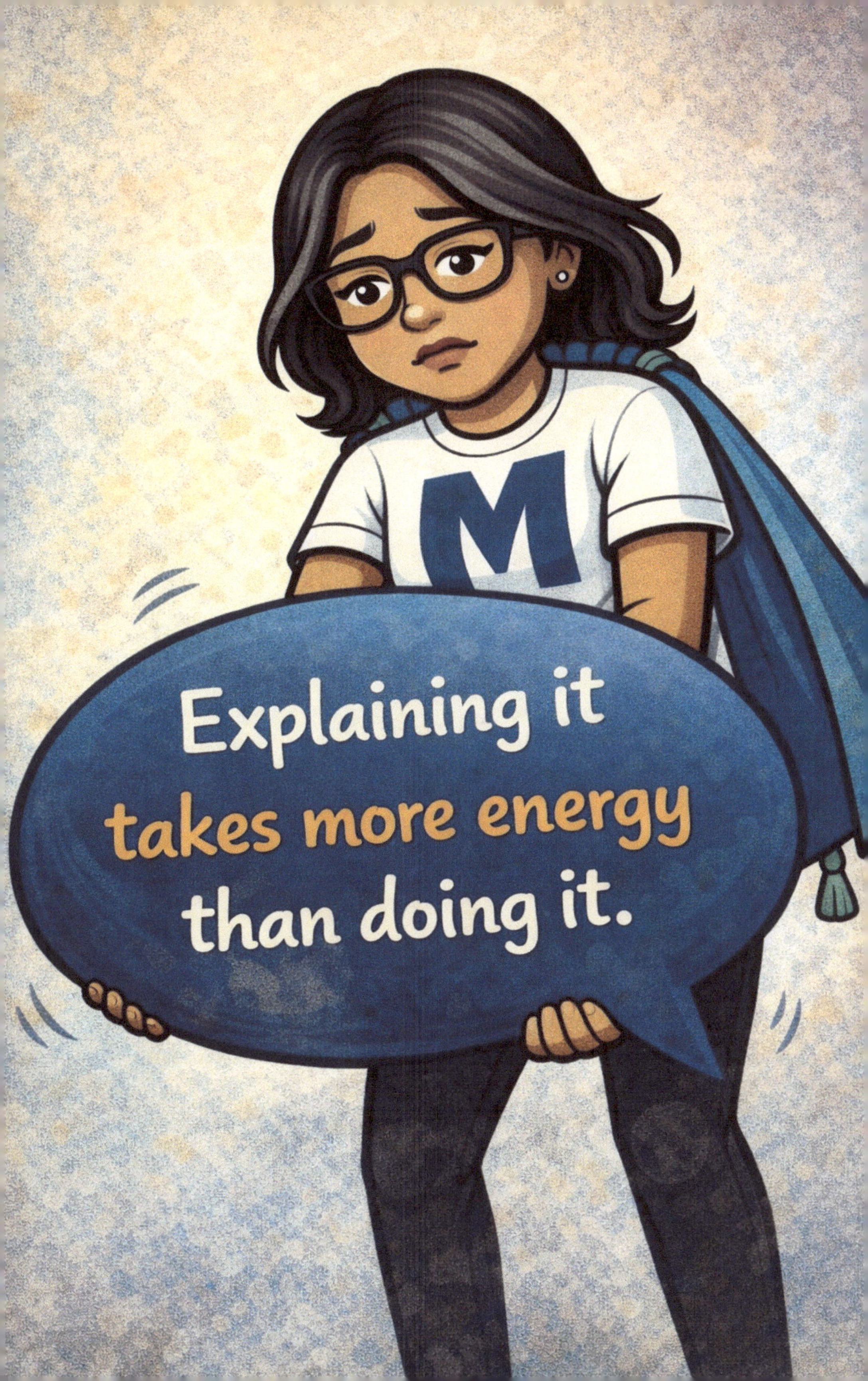
M
Explaining it takes more energy than doing it.

Burnout doesn't wait until life slows down.
It doesn't wait for the right moment.

It arrives quietly,
even while you're still showing up every day.

And by the time you notice it,
you've been carrying it far longer than you realize.

I ran out

before I was allowed to.

You were never meant to carry it all alone.
Some things are always optional.

Some things can be set down,
even if it feels unfamiliar at first.

You are allowed to loosen your grip.

Not everything is yours to carry.

Real help doesn't need instructions.
It sees what's happening.
It notices what's needed.

It steps in without waiting to be asked.

It makes room where there wasn't any,
and eases what you didn't have words for.

Help doesn't ask.

It notices.

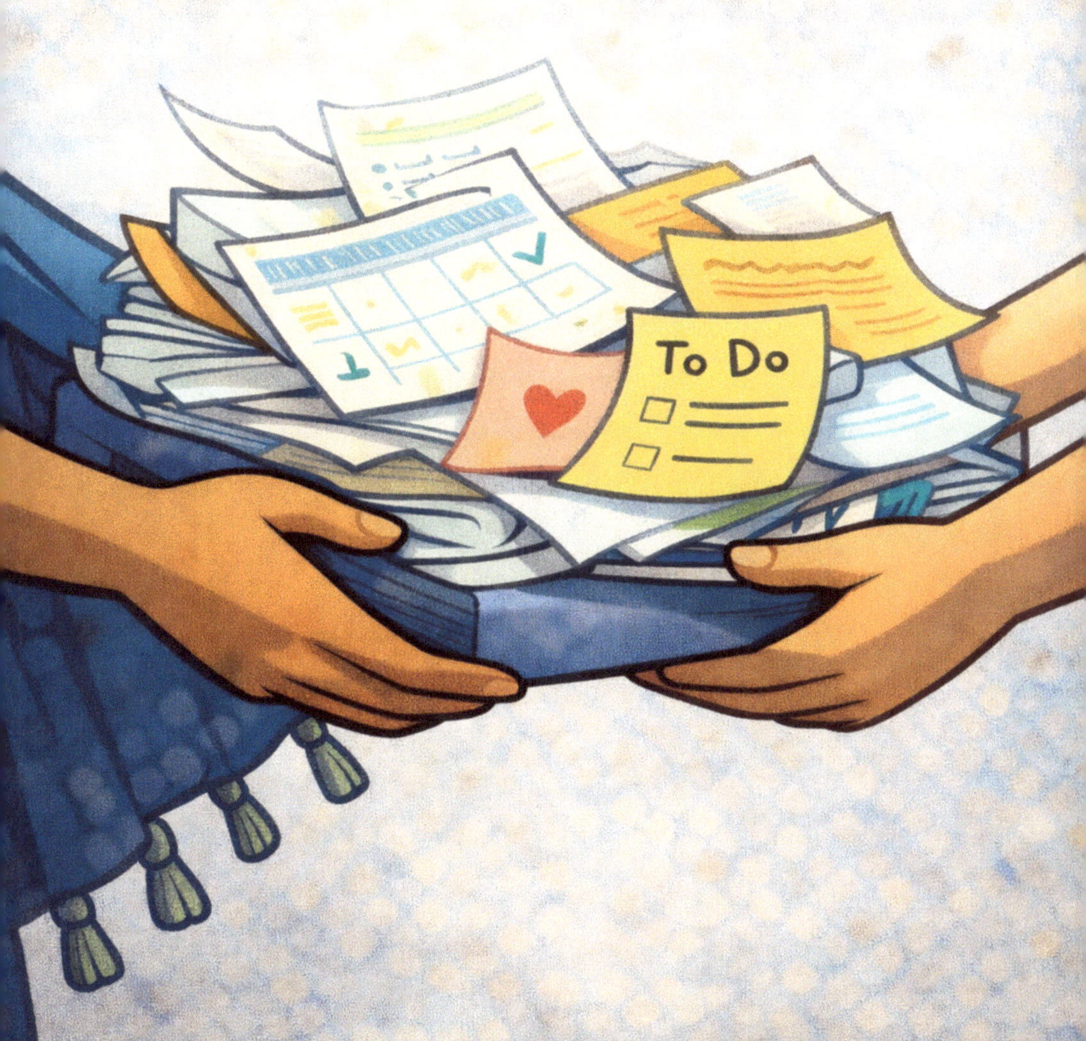

The goal is never perfection.

Perfection was never the measure of a life well lived.

The goal is living.

It is being here.

It is showing up for the life that is happening
right now.

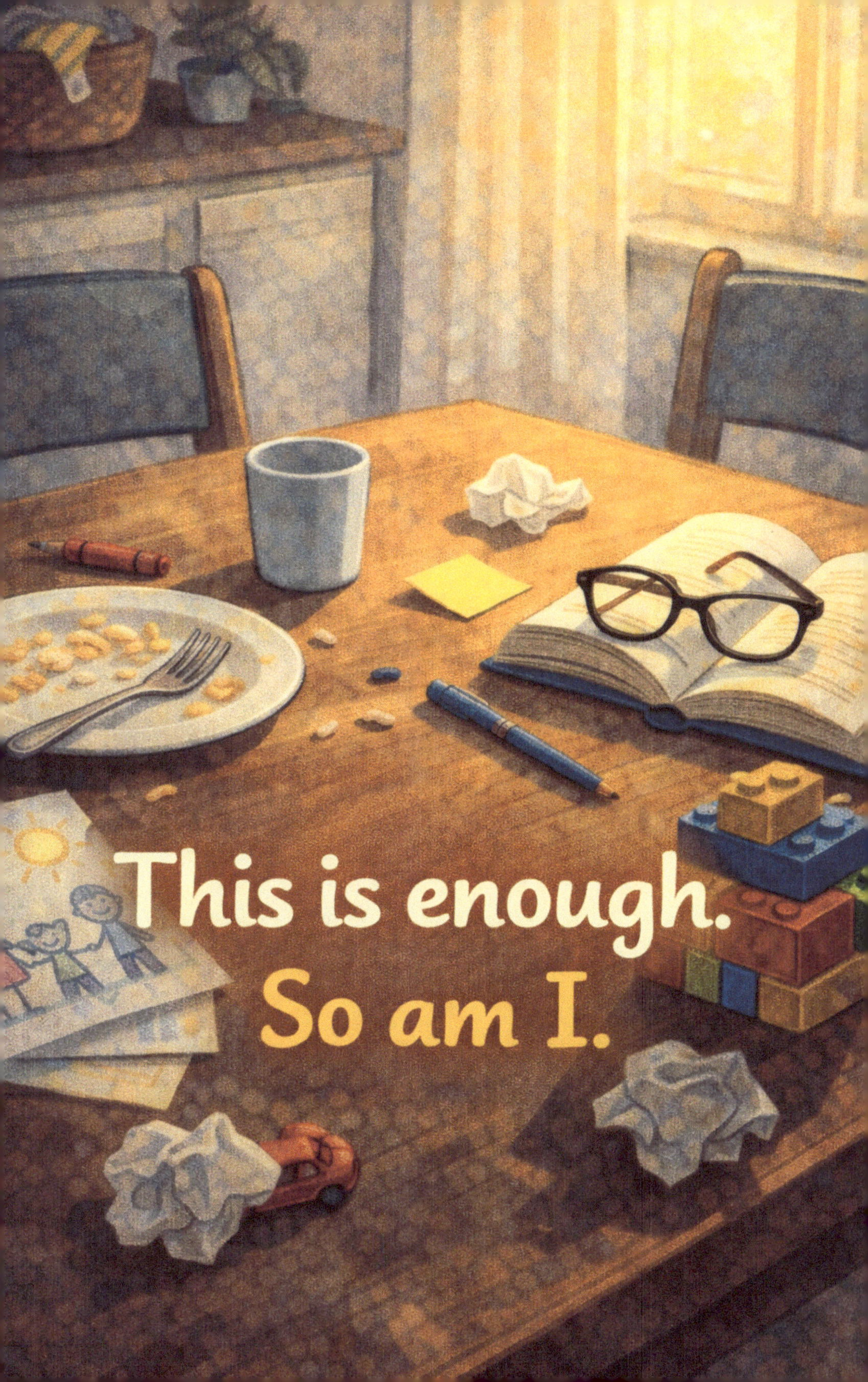
This is enough.
So am I.

You don't need to disappear to deserve rest.
You don't need to earn quiet by doing more.

Rest belongs to you too.
You can choose yourself without guilt.

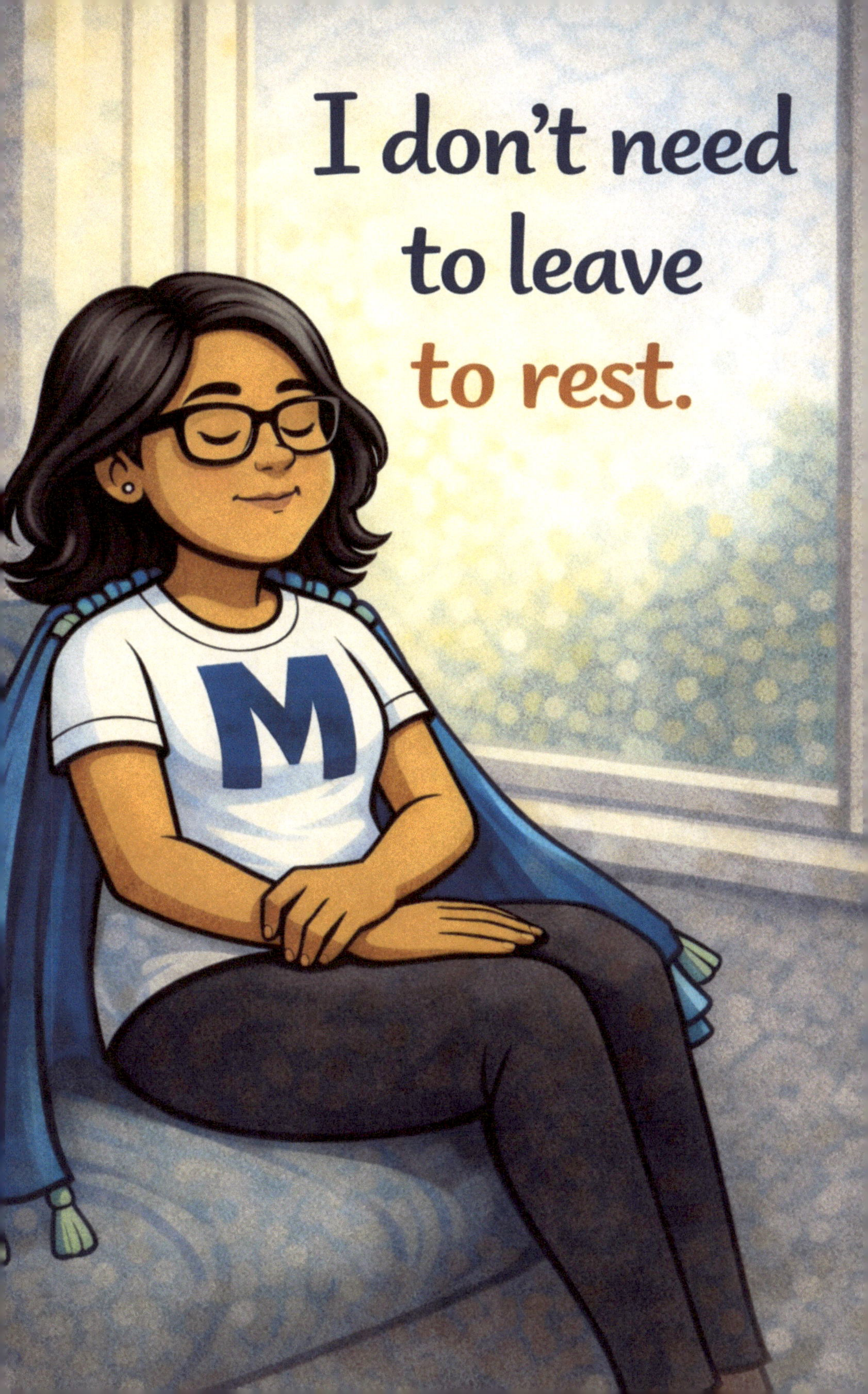
I don't need
to leave
to rest.

There's nothing wrong with you.
You are not failing.

You are carrying what no one named,
the things that live in your mind
long before they ever become visible.

Nothing is wrong with you.
You are just holding too much.

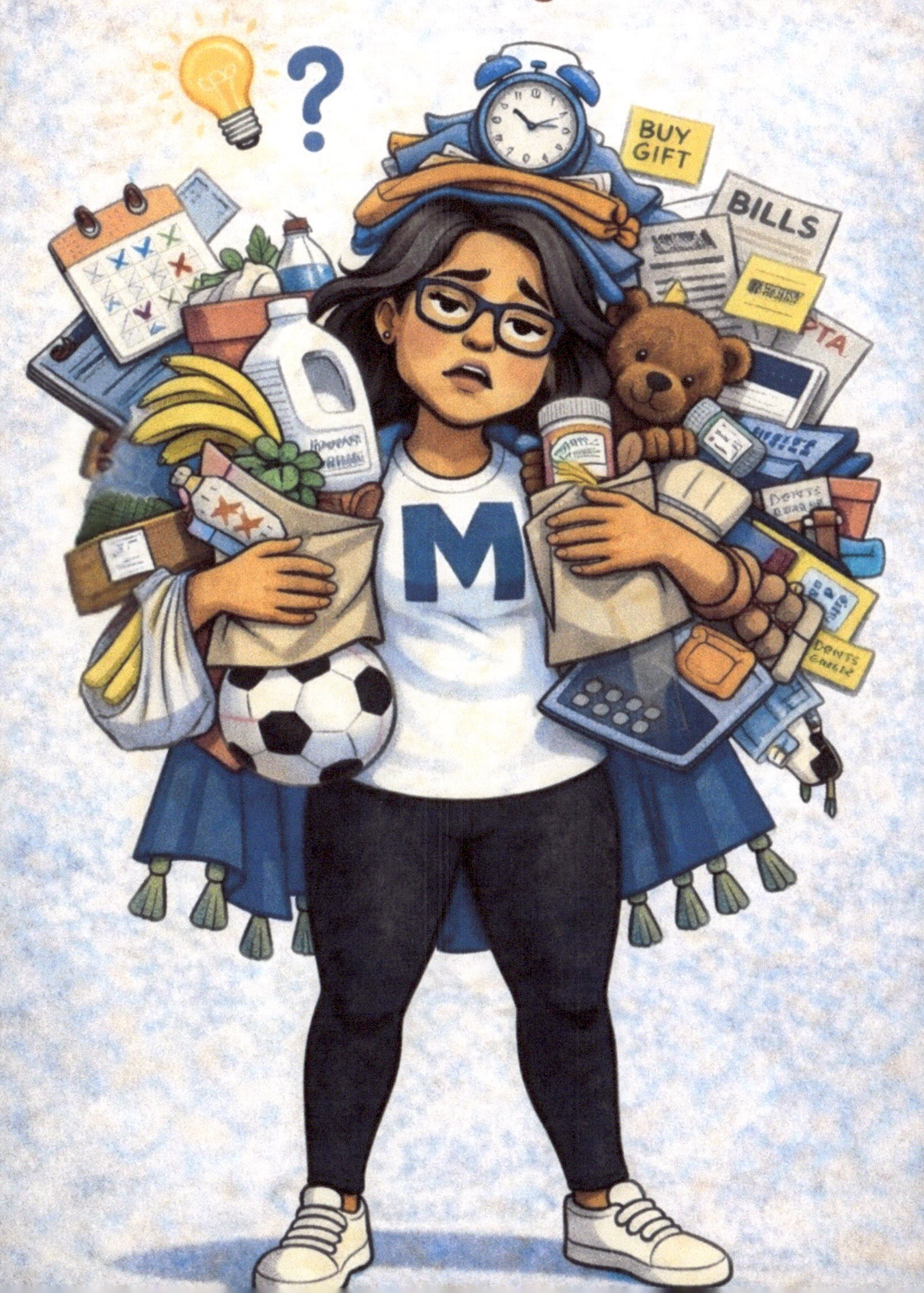

You are not tired for no reason.
You are not failing.

You are doing real, unseen work —
and you have been carrying it for a long time.

If you feel even a little lighter now,
let that matter.

You don't have to earn rest.
You don't have to finish everything first.

What you have done matters
more than you know.

And you don't have to carry it
the same way anymore. ♡

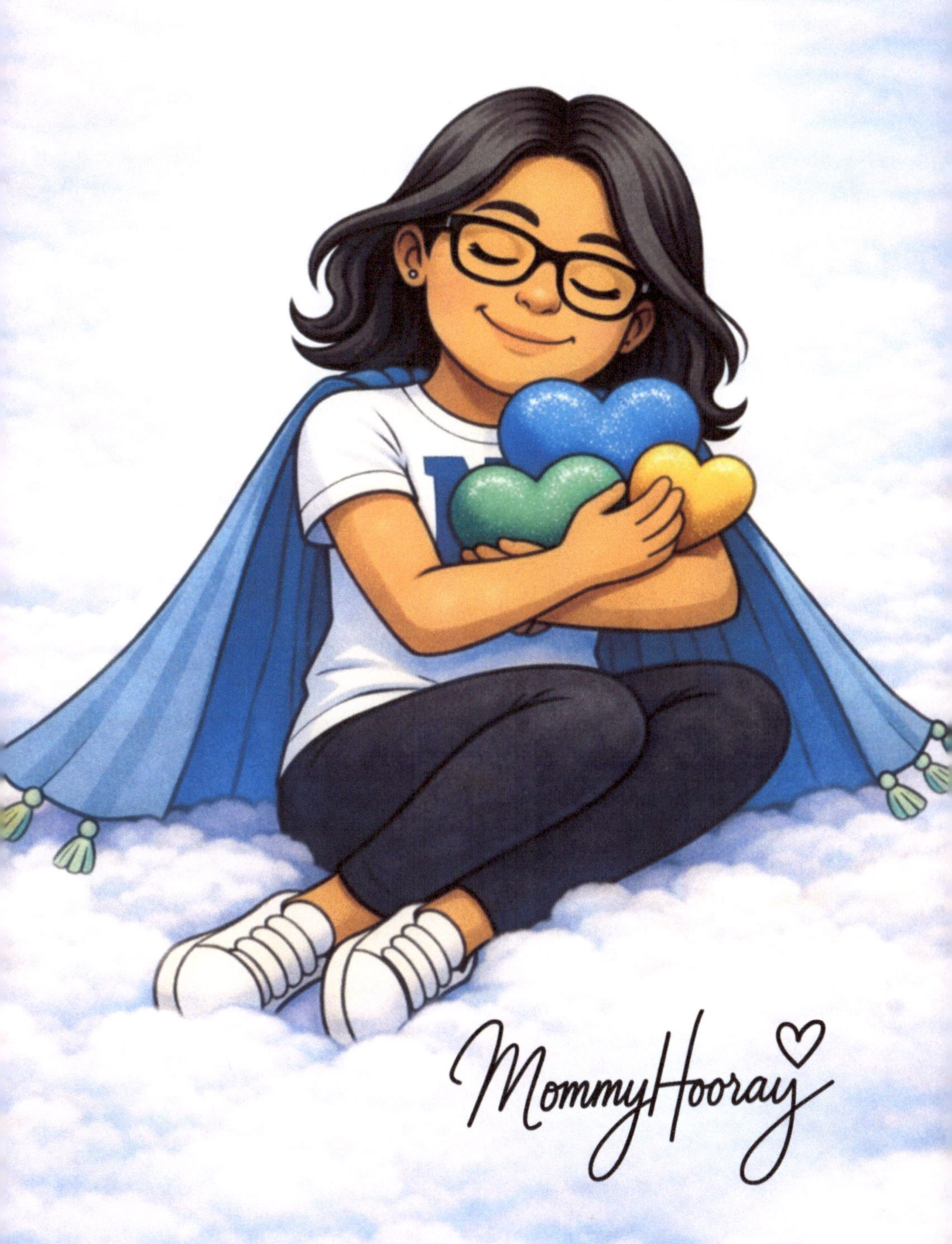
MommyHooray

Also by MommyHooray

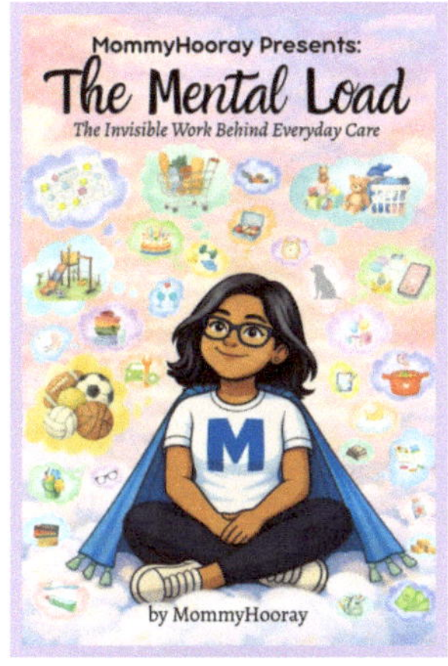

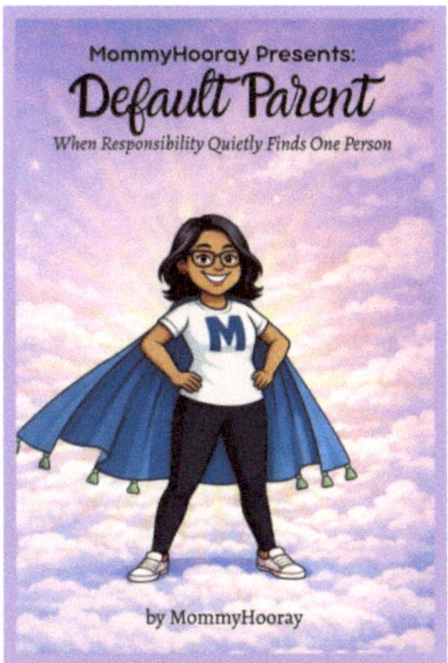

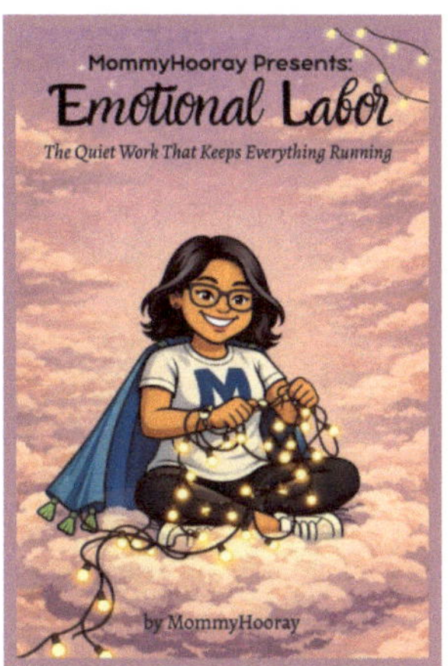

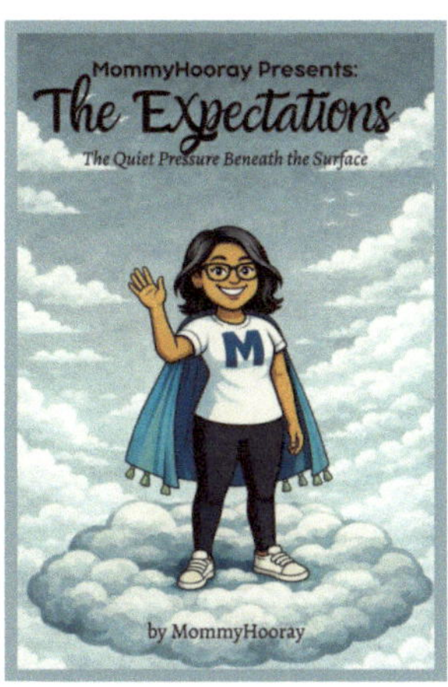

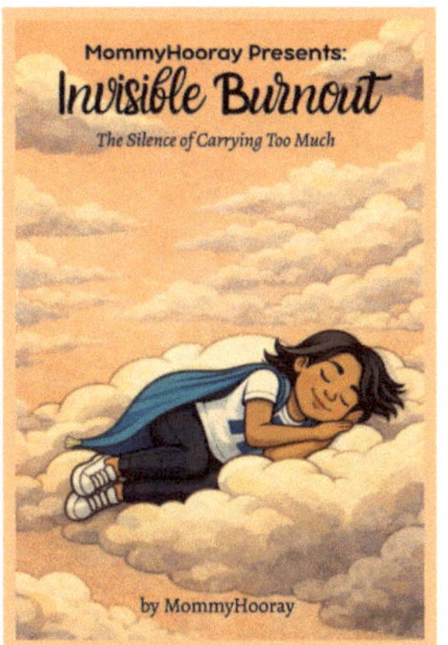

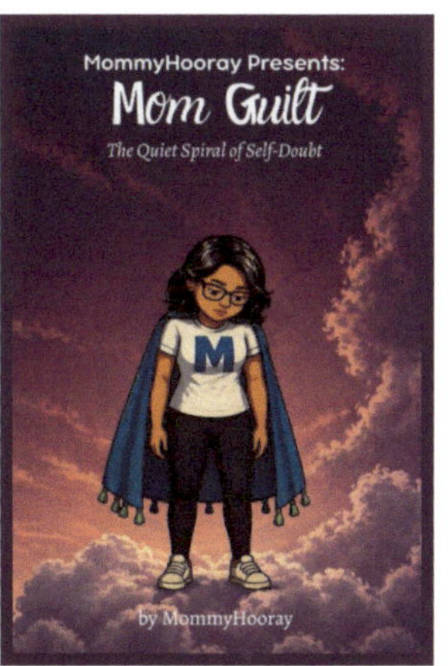

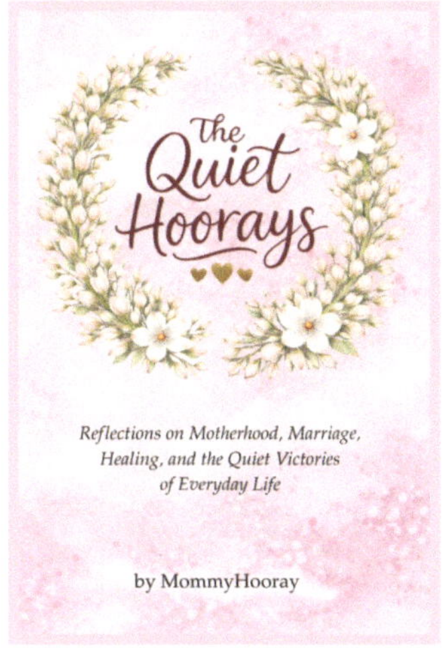

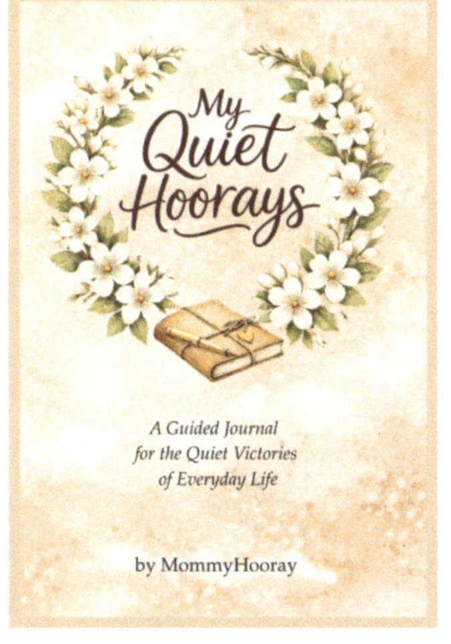

... and more!

From My Heart to Yours

Write something meaningful
for the person who will cherish this book, or for yourself.

Today's Date: ________________

May this page find you again, years from now.

www.ingramcontent.com/pod-product-compliance
Lightning Source LLC
LaVergne TN
LVHW052300100826
845147LV00001B/99

9781972071403